LEARN ALL ABOUT OSTEOARTHRITIS PAIN TREATMENT & PREVENTION
Authentic Medical Facts for Patients

<u>(Large Print)</u>

Dr A Mitra MBBS, MD, DMI

Disclaimer:

The information provided in this book is correct to the best of my knowledge. However, it is not a substitute for the professional advice. This book provides information only and how the reader uses it is their choice. The author / publishers are not liable for inappropriate use of the information by any reader.

CONTENT

- How is OA treated?
- Which treatment is best for OA?
- How can you treat OA without medications?
- What is the role of Rest in treatment of OA?
- How does weight reduction help in OA?
- How does Exercise help in OA?
- What are Orthoses?
- What types of Orthotic devices are there?
- Are there any supportive or assistive devices available for use at home?
- How can I select the most

appropriate assistive / supportive device ?

- What is the role of Vitamins in OA?

- Can applying heat /cold pack help in OA?

- What is TENS and how does it help in OA?

- What is the role of patient education in OA ?

- What sort of psycho-social support can help?

- What is the role of Alternative Therapies in OA?

- What types of Mediciations can help with OA ?

- What is the role of Nonsteroidal anti–inflammatory (NSAIDS) drugs ?
- How does creams, gels and patches available for pain relief work in OA?
- What is the role of Joint Injections in OA?
- How does Surgery help in OA?
- What are the complications of OA?
- How to Prevent OA?
- How to live well even with OA?
- **References**

Author Biography

Dr A Mitra is a medical doctor registered with the Australian Health Practitioners Regulation Agency (AHPRA.gov.au).

He had his medical education in India (MBBS, MD). Then he did further education in Medical Informatics from UK (DMI). Subsequently, he moved over to Australia where he had been working in the health system after completing the certification examination conducted by Australian Medical Council.

At present, he works as a locum doctor in Australia. He spends his free-time reading, writing and painting.

Preface

Today as medical practitioners we have become busier than ever before. As a result, we are unable to do justice to our patients by not being able to answer all their queries and questions.

Consequently, the apprehensive patient turns to Mr. Google to find the answers. Unfortunately, the Internet is unregulated and full of misleading information about medicine. This has led to many dangerous consequences for patients.

Since the time when I did my post graduate diploma in Medical Informatics many years ago, I have been keen on using the knowledge to benefit my patients by creating authentic easy to read medical information booklets for patients. Writing this book is part of my humble contribution to the welfare of the patients.

Hope that every reader finds something in this book, which benefits them. If so, I will feel that, my time and effort have come to some good use.

This will make me more motivated to write similar books on other conditions.

Dr A Mitra
August 2014

OSTEO–ARTHRITIS

What is Osteoarthritis (OA)?

Osteoarthritis (OA) is a common type of arthritis in which there is a slow thinning of cartilage material in the joints.

It is also commonly called arthritis.

It is a gradually progressive condition involving different joints.

How does OA develop?

The bones that meet at a joint normally tend not to rub against each other, mainly because these are typically protected by a rubber like substance known as cartilage.

In individuals with osteoarthritis, the cartilage material wears down, and the bone surfaces rub against one another causing discomfort.

At times, the bones can also develop projections referred to as spurs.

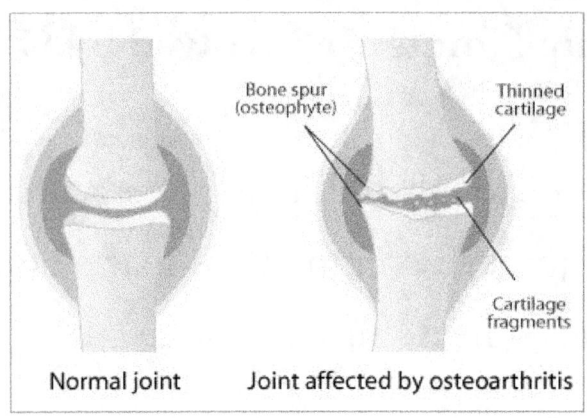

Normal joint   Joint affected by osteoarthritis

Bone spur (osteophyte)

Thinned cartilage

Cartilage fragments

Which joints are involved by OA?

Even though OA may affect virtually any joint, it commonly impacts on the hands, knees, hips, and spine.

How long does OA last?

Osteoarthritis is a long-term problem which progressively gets worse with time.

Then again, there are many methods that may slow down its advancement as well as reduce discomfort.

The medical diagnosis of OA is the initial component of making sure that the best treatments for osteoarthritis are utilized.

What types of OA are there?

You will find two principal types of osteoarthritis which have different causative factors.

Idiopathic osteoarthritis

Idiopathic OA has basically no recognizable trigger.

It is usually localized (limited to just one or two joints) or generalised (found in three or more joints).

Secondary osteoarthritis

Secondary OA is a result of some other underlying problem which can be any of the following:

- a joint accident,
- collection of calcium within the joint,
- another bone and joint illnesses (like, rheumatoid arthritis),
- or even a medical problem like

diabetes mellitus.

What are the common symptoms of OA?

The signs and symptoms of OA generally start after age forty and may differ substantially from one individual to another. The include the following:

Pain

The most common indication of OA is joint soreness, which is much worse with exercise and is also reduced by rest.

In serious situations, the pain could

also manifest while resting or even at nighttime.

The pain sensation generally starts close to the involved joint; then again, occasionally, the discomfort could be referred to some other locations.

For instance, the pain of OA of the hip joint could possibly appear as part of the knee.

Joint parts impacted by OA could be sensitive to touch.

The degree of pain may become

constant as time passes.

Any sort of abrupt increases in the degree of discomfort may suggest some new injury or an underlying disease such as gout.

Stiffness

Morning stiffness is a typical manifestation of OA.

This stiffness generally resolves within thirty minutes of rising from bed.

However, it could reoccur during the

day at times of inactivity.

Many individuals notice a change in symptoms linked with the weather conditions.

Inflammation (swelling)

Osteoarthritis could produce a kind of joint swelling known as an effusion.

This is the result of the collection of excessive liquid within the joint space.

Crackling or grating feeling (crepitus)

Activity involving joints troubled by OA may cause a crackling or grating feeling called crepitus.

This feeling probably develops as a result of roughening of the ordinarily smooth surfaces on the inside of the joint.

Bony outgrowths (osteophytes)

OA in many cases leads to outgrowths of bone known as osteophytes or bone spurs.

These types of bony protuberances

may be felt below your skin near joint parts.

These usually increase with time.

Symptoms in specified joints

Osteoarthritis does not impact all joints uniformly.

The problem typically impacts the fingers, knees, hips, and spine.

It seldom affects the elbow, wrist, and ankle.

In addition, it often impacts joint parts on a single side of the body differently in contrast to on the opposite side.

Common symptoms in any joint begins with one or more of the following:

- Pain
- Stiffness
- Difficult joint movements

What happens over time with OA?

OA is a continuous ongoing problem with episodic worsening.

Over time condition usually gets worse.

However proper joint care decrease discomfort and allows people to stay on physically active.

Some believe that it may possibly slow down the deterioration of the condition.

What are the Risk Factors for OA?

A multitude of causes can increase the chance of getting OA.

The majority of individuals with OA have one or more of these risk factors.

Age

Getting old is probably the most potent causative factor for OA.

The problem seldom happens in individuals younger than age forty.

However, at least eighty per cent of individuals over age fifty-five already have X-ray signs associated with the condition.

Then again, not every individual with OA on an X-ray suffers from joint pain or some other joint difficulty.

Gender

For unknown reasons, females are approximately two and three times more susceptible compared to males to develop OA.

Overweight

Individuals who are heavy have higher risk of getting OA.

Weight reduction could lower this particular risk.

Occupation

OA of the knee joint appears to have been linked with particular jobs that involve repeated squatting and kneeling, such as cotton production, loading dock jobs, shipyard work, and woodworking.

OA of the hip joint happens to be connected with farm work, construction work, plus other works that involve lifting of heavy items, prolonged standing, or walking long distances daily.

Sports

The danger of OA is enhanced in those who indulge in specific sporting events, such as wrestling, boxing, pitching in baseball, bicycling, parachuting, cricket, gymnastics, ballet dancing, soccer, and football.

In comparison, running does not seem to enhance the chance of OA.

Family history

In several instances, OA can run in family members.

Hereditary studies have not really revealed any single gene responsible for OA.

So it could be possible that a large number of genes make little contributions each.

This information suggests that it is not possible to discover a genetic testing for OA in the immediate future.

How is OA diagnosed?

Generally, there is no constant sign, symptom, or testing which can identify OA.

As an alternative, the particular diagnosis of OA is dependent upon consideration of a number of points, such as the typical observable manifestations of OA plus the outcomes of laboratory investigations and X-rays.

X-rays are usually a good choice for monitoring the state of OA in the long run.

However, x-rays may seem normal, especially during the initial phases of OA.

Other kinds of imaging investigations, like Ultrasound and Magnetic Resonance Imaging (MRI), could be employed to identify destruction of cartilage material, ligaments, and tendons, that may not be observed on x-ray.

What is the course of OA?

Osteoarthritis usually gets worse gradually with time, even though it may stabilize in some cases.

In those individuals whose pain and joint stiffness get worse with time, there is in most cases periodic deteriorations (deterioration, then improvement for a time period).

Some individuals with osteoarthritis are in a position to function routinely in spite of discomfort whilst others could possibly face hardships with even basic activities due to the pain.

Physical exercise can help to protect against reduction in strength and also could lower the possibilities of getting handicapped in the long run.

How is OA treated?

OA is treated with a combination of different types of treatments which includes the following:

- Non–medication remedies
- Medication treatments
- Occasionally surgical treatments

Which treatment is best for OA?

For OA treatment, methods are individualized according to patient's condition and therefore, may differ from one patient to another.

When deciding on treatment the following issues are considered.

- Severity of problem
- Type of joints involved
- Effect of specific intervention on individual patient

How can you treat OA without medications?

Non-medication treatment is the first option in treatment of OA.

It can improve OA symptoms temporarily.

These include the following:

- Rest
- Weight loss
- Physical therapy
- Exercise programs
- Orthoses

What is the role of Rest in treatment of OA?

OA symptoms are usually worsened by excessive activities.

These are also improved temporarily by rest.

However, total inactivity is harmful as it causes loss in muscle tissue plus increases joint stiffness.

When pain increases, temporary rest for 12 to 24 hours is beneficial.

After that you can return to regular functions but avoid excessive activities.

How does weight reduction help in OA?

Obesity is associated with OA of the knee joint.

Weight reduction lessens this particular risk of developing OA.

However, it is not known yet if it decreases the worsening of already affected joints.

Current medical evidence reveals that weight reduction is specially effective in lowering hip and knee joint pain.

How does Exercise help in OA?

Physiotherapy consists of exercise programs.

This improves flexibility by strengthening the muscles surrounding the joints affected by OA.

This in turn lessens pain and improves functioning of the joints.

What are Orthoses?

Orthoses are specialized accessories that safeguard joint functionality by keeping the joints aligned properly which in return lowers symptoms.

What types of Orthotic devices are there?

Orthotic footwear are padded shoes to decrease strain on the OA joints.

Splints are used to immobilize the OA joints.

They can be used throughout the day

and also night and they help to reduce pain and swelling.

Braces are used to support unsteady joints.

Are there any supportive or assistive devices available for use at home?

Supportive device (also called Mobility Aids) can be used at home.

They include walking-sticks, walkers, electric-powered seat lifts, elevated commode chairs, bathtub and shower bars.

These intend to lower the strain on OA joints and thereby assist in carrying out day-to-day activities.

How can I select the most appropriate assistive / supportive device ?

Your physiotherapist can help you in this matter by evaluating the seriousness of the problem and then recommend a suitable assistive equipment based upon the severity and location of your OA.

What is the role of Vitamins in OA?

The advantage of specific vitamins in joint wellness continues to be investigated and there is no clean verdict as of today.

The information that researchers have found out so far is that OA is much less likely to deteriorate in individuals who have a high dietary consumption of vitamin C (ascorbic acid) and a higher diet content as well as higher blood amounts of vitamin D.

Can applying heat /cold pack help in OA?

Heat and cold therapies – reduce OA difficulties like pain and stiffness.

Heat therapy reduces pain and stiffness in osteoarthritic joints.

Heat can be applied to the joints using hot packs, hot water bottles, heating pads, or electrically heated mittens.

It is vital to prevent burning up your skin when making use of heat therapy.

To prevent skin burns, hot water bottles need to be filled up using warm, not boiling hot water.

Heating pads should always be put on a timer and applied for no longer than twenty minutes at any given time.

The heating pad may be re-used after twenty minutes of no use.

Cold therapy reduces pain in arthritic joints and lowers muscle spasms.

Cold can be utilized for brief

durations making use of ice packs or coolant sprays.

Individuals having specific health problems, for example Raynaud phenomenon, must avoid using cold therapy.

What is TENS and how does it help in OA?

TENS stands for Transcutaneous Electrical Nerve Stimulation (TENS).

A TENS device gives a light electric current to your skin thereby exciting nerve fibers in the skin that intervene in the sending of pain signals from the OA joint.

The application of TENS as a means of osteoarthritis therapy is at the present moment debatable.

Certain research reports have found out that individuals who make use of TENS for arthritis of the knee have diminished knee pain, an improved capacity to flex the knee, and also a diminished time period of early-morning stiffness.

Conversely, some other research report found out that TENS was no more beneficial in reducing pain compared to medication naproxen or even a placebo.

What is the role of patient education in OA ?

Patient understanding of their condition is helpful to sufferers for a variety of reasons.

OA discomfort could lead you to become miserable, reliant on other people for assistance, and in many cases really feel depressed.

All these issues could lessen your enthusiasm to continue with OA therapy.

On the other hand, by simply learning more about OA, you can actually get more focused with your own personal therapy.

It is essential for you to talk about the alternatives for treating OA and also the consequences of OA upon everyday living.

Additionally, you should discuss the possible methods for the managing of the particular restrictions imposed by OA with your professional medical physician.

A number of researches indicate that psychological and social assistance could be as successful as medication treatment for the lowering of the discomfort of OA.

What sort of psycho-social support can help?

Support can be obtained in a variety of ways.

For instance, it's possible to benefit simply by developing a friendly support circle or perhaps join an online support group.

Even where possible interactions or even though active involvement with a specialized OA support group is useful.

Information regarding some of the support groups in your country can easily be found on internet search.

What is the role of Alternative Therapies in OA?

Quite a few different remedies have now been examined to ascertain whether they have any sort of result on OA.

Nutritional supplements

Glucosamine and chondroitin are nutritional supplements that have received plenty of focus because of their possible benefits in lowering discomfort along with delaying the advancement of OA.

Glucosamine

One preparation of Glucosamine called Glucosamine Hydrochloride when compared with placebo in a well-designed research ended up being not much more effective in reducing OA pain or even in boosting joint function.

However, it is quite possible that another preparation type could be beneficial and therefore, further research is being conducted by scientists.

Current medical opinion is that glucosamine really does not seem to slow down the decline of OA in the long run.

There are a few undesirable side effects of glucosamine, for example, it must not be tried by patients who are sensitive to seafood.

Chondroitin

Chondroitin used by itself may produce a minimal advantage for people who have OA.

There are not any major adverse side effects of chondroitin.

Also the mixture of glucosamine and chondroitin sulfate has not proven to be any better when compared with placebo for pain reduction or even for functioning improvement in individuals with OA of the knee joint.

Traditional Chinese Medicine

Different aspects of traditional Chinese Medicine, such as natural herbs as well as Acupuncture therapy, could help manage the OA discomfort in some cases, even though the advantages of these types of treatments have not yet been verified in major, well-organized scientific research.

Reumalex, willow bark, stinging nettle, Articulin-F, devil's claw, extract of soybean and avocado unsaponifiables (ASU), and Phytodolor may possibly lower OA pain, whereas some other herbal plants and mixtures like for example Eazmov, Gitadyl, or even ginger extract are perhaps not helpful.

If you intend on the use of herbal

supplements, speak with your professional medical service provider.

Capsaicin cream

Many individuals report having a reduction of OA discomfort after they apply products that contain capsaicin, the active chemical found in hot chili peppers.

Capsaicin diminishes a pain-causing chemical located in nerve endings and in addition lowers the OA pain by about thirty per cent in some cases.

Forty percent individuals report having side-effects when applying capsaicin cream, which includes burning, stinging, and inflammation of the skin and particularly the eye.

Others

Using things like dimethylsulfoxide (DMSO) or making use of low-power laser light, copper bracelets, or magnets are usually of uncertain results.

Chiropractic manipulation, acupressure, biofeedback, and

homeopathy are widespread.

However, according to current evidence these actually have unverified effects with regards to OA discomfort.

What types of Mediciations can help with OA?

Medication treatments are an essential part of the OA plan for treatment.

Various kinds of medications are on the market.

Pain Reduction Medications

Analgesics

Analgesics decrease pain, however have no impact on joint inflammation.

These types of medicines are usually suggested whenever OA pain does not get better with non- pharmacologic methods.

Medications within this class consist of acetaminophen (Paracetamol) and also opioid (narcotic) analgesics.

Acetaminophen (Paracetamol) can reduce mild to moderate OA pain.

To prevent the harmful but rare side effects of kidney as well as liver damage because of acetaminophen, it is essential to adhere to dosing recommendations and stay away from consuming too much quantities of alcoholic beverages.

Narcotic analgesics

The pain due to abrupt, intense worsening of OA could need intervention using narcotic analgesics such as codeine.

Narcotics need to be used only for brief periods as they can be habit-forming.

They could be most successful when

used along with nonsteroidal antiinflammatory drugs (NSAIDs).

Narcotics may be also used in combination with acetaminophen .

What is the role of Nonsteroidal anti-inflammatory (**NSAIDS**) drugs ?

NSAIDs medications reduce pain and decrease joint inflammation. Most of the non-prescription products which are for sale to treat OA pain are usually NSAIDs.

These types of medications are commonly suggested before the analgesics for individuals that have OA plus signs of joint swelling (inflammation).

They are additionally suggested for many people with non-inflammatory OA who actually are not getting sufficient pain alleviation with simple analgesics.

How does creams, gels and patches available for pain relief work in OA?

Following a particularly physically active week your joints may ache even with your regular osteoarthritis pain medication. In such a situation perhaps you may want to get an over the counter joint cream or patch that claims to decrease the pain sensation.

Topical pain medications are absorbed into your skin layer. The most popular options are creams or gels which you massage on the skin surface on top of your aching joint parts. Some varieties are available in the form of a spray or a patch that adheres on your skin. Because the ingredients are soaked up through the skin, the majority of topical pain medications are ideally applied to joint parts, which are near the skin's surface, for instance, the joints in your hands and knees.

Feedback can vary with regard to usefulness of non-prescription topical pain treatments. Even though many individuals claim these kinds of products help to temporarily relieve their joint pain, clinical research shows only minor advantages. A couple of products work virtually not any better than placebo in reducing osteoarthritis discomfort.

Do not use local pain-killer on cracked or irritated skin area or even in combination with a heating pad or bandage.

The active compounds in nonprescription applicable pain medications can contain:

Capsaicin

Capsaicin induces a burning feeling you correlate with chili peppers. Capsaicin products empty your nerve cells of a substance which is essential for transmitting pain signals. Use of capsaicin products could make the skin burn or sting. However, this particular discomfort typically reduces in a couple of weeks of regular usage. Wash your hands properly after every single application and abstain from touching your eyes and mucous membranes. You could use latex gloves when putting on the cream.

Salicylates

Salicylates creams have the same pain-relieving chemical which is present in aspirin. Salicylates seem to be a lot more reliable for muscle aches, whereas capsaicin products are usually used in pain linked with damaged nerves – such as postherpetic neuralgia. If you are allergic to aspirin or are using blood thinners, consult with your medical professional prior to using topical treatments, which contain salicylates.

Counterirritants

Compounds like menthol and camphor create a feeling of hot or cold that may momentarily supersede your ability to feel your joint disease pain.

NSAID cream

Oral medications that contain nonsteroidal anti-inflammatory drugs (NSAIDs) are a popular treatment plan for osteoarthritis, but they can irritate the stomach. A lot of medical professionals suggest NSAID creams or gels simply because they possess a reduced likelihood of gastric irritation. Various researches show a large number of NSAID creams and gels work as well as their oral counterparts for mild to moderate discomfort, particularly in locations where joints are close to skin, for example, in finger joints.

Lidocaine Patches

In a few cases, physicians might recommend patches that contain a numbing medicine, like lidocaine, for joint aches. Patches are put onto the skin over the painful joint for twelve-hour periods.

What is the role of Joint Injections in OA?

Two kinds of injection therapy can be used for those that have osteoarthritis pain:

- glucocorticoid (steroid) injections and
- injections of a liquid called hyaluronate.

Glucocorticoid (steroid) injections

Glucocorticoids could reduce joint inflammation and could very well reduce OA discomfort after being injected into arthritic joints.

Glucocorticoid injections could possibly be suggested for those who have OA limited to a couple of joints and additionally who continue to get serious pain in spite of the using NSAIDs.

Glucocorticoid injections might additionally be suggested for people who have OA but are unable to use NSAIDs.

Joint injections come with little

unwanted side effects.

However, some individuals experience having a short flare-up of osteoarthritis symptoms following an injection.

Generally there can also be a limited chance of joint infection.

Glucocorticoids may perhaps harm some joint parts if injected continuously.

That is why, physicians suggest a maximum of three or four injection therapy each year for every individual weight–bearing joint like the knee joint.

Hyaluronate injections

Typical joint fluid is made up of a substantial amount of hyaluronate, that allows the joint fluid to be smooth.

Artificial hyaluronates could be injected inside the knee joint for treating OA.

Following the injection, pain

reduction may perhaps continue for many months.

Hyaluronan (Hyalgan) and hylan–GF–20 (Synvisc) are a couple of products, which may be used and seem to be very much the same in their outcomes.

These types of substances are typically injected into the knee joint.

However their use in some other joint is actually being researched.

Joint inflammation has sometimes

developed following this type of injection.

Just like steroid treatments, there is also a tiny chance of infection.

Therefore, should you experience significant joint pain shortly after an injection, contact your medical care provider instantly.

Hyaluronate injections are usually restricted to individuals with OA who are unable to use NSAIDs or who do not attain good relief of pain with these.

Individuals waiting for joint surgery may possibly gain from such treatments.

Colchicine

This particular medication is usually suggested for those with inflamed OA, which fails to get better with the help of non–pharmacologic treatments and NSAlDs.

A doctor will probably suggest colchicine for those who get repeated flare up of OA, which is resistant to various other treatment options.

Hydroxychloroquine

Hydroxychloroquine (Plaquenil) shows immune-modulating benefits, which minimize the joint inflammation associated with OA in some cases.

This particular medication could be suggested for individuals with serious inflammation related to OA as well as for those individuals who have bone tissue destruction in connection with OA.

How does Surgery help in OA?

Surgical treatment is normally restricted to extreme osteoarthritis, which substantially restricts an individual's lifestyle and also fails to respond to various other OA treatment options.

Conversely, surgical procedure is usually recommended prior to OA triggered additional complications like muscle mass thinning plus joint deformities.

In addition, individuals who go

through operative procedures should really be in the best achievable fitness and must be ready for the rehabilitation shortly after a operative procedure.

The types of surgical procedures include the following:

Arthroscopy and joint irrigation

The advantage associated with the arthroscopic surgical procedure in individuals with osteoarthritis is actually marked by controversy.

Having said that, a particular selection of individuals with OA may perhaps really benefit from arthroscopy.

Then again, individuals with considerable OA are a lot more likely to gain from some other kinds of surgical procedures.

Realignment

Surgical treatment can be used in order to realign bones and other joint structures, which have been out of alignment as a result of long lasting OA.

With regard to the knee joint, realignment could adjust weight-bearing to healthier cartilage in order to reduce OA pain.

This particular kind of alignment could possibly be suggested for the younger healthier individuals as an alternative to joint replacement operation.

Fusion

Surgical procedures can be used to permanently join several bones together with each other inside the joint.

This could be suggested for the seriously affected joint parts for which joint replacement surgery is not necessarily recommended.

Fusion may well be proposed for joints of the wrist and ankle and for the tiny joint parts of fingers and toes.

Joint replacement

Surgical treatment can be used to replace an affected joint with an artificial joint.

The most frequent reason behind having joint replacement surgery is pain that is not managed through a combination of non-pharmacologic and medication treatments.

Joint replacement surgery significantly alleviates discomfort in individuals having serious OA of the hip or knee, and this particular benefit seems to persist not less than three years.

Conversely, it could take as many as twelve months before the advantages of joint replacement surgery end up being truly evident.

Cartilage grafting

Surgical treatment can be used to transplant new cartilage tissue into damaged areas of cartilage.

The benefits of cartilage grafting in arthritic joints are being researched.

Cartilage grafting is likely to be most useful when the cartilage problem is limited to a very small section which is flanked by healthy cartilage.

Current approaches are not useful for those who have large sections of flimsy or absent cartilage material.

What are the complications of OA?

- Reduced mobility
- Chronic Pain
- Infection following surgical interventions

How to Prevent OA?

Stopping Osteoarthritis

It is impossible to stop OA completely.

Then again, you may well be capable of limiting your own chance of developing it by averting injuries plus trying to keep healthy.

Start looking after your joints

Perform some routine physical exercise, however, do not put too much strain on your joints, especially your hips, knees and the joints in your hands.

Skip exercises which put stress upon your joint parts and causes them to carry an unreasonable weight, for example, running and weight training.

As a substitute, perform activities like swimming and cycling, whereby all of your joint parts are better supported, and the burden is much manageable.

Attempt to uphold ideal posture always, and steer clear of remaining in the exact same posture for a long time.

When you work on a desk, ensure that your seat is actually at the proper height and also take frequent breaks to move around.

Always keep the muscles healthy.

Your muscular tissues assist in maintaining your own joint parts, therefore, having powerful muscle tissue can help your joints remain healthy too.

Consider exercising for not less than

150 minutes (2 hours and 30 minutes) with reasonable intensity aerobic activity (i.e. cycling or fast walking) each week to develop your muscle vitality.

Work out should really be enjoyable, so do what you get pleasure from, then again, try to avoid overburden on the joints.

Reduce body weight in case you're heavy.

Remaining overweight can make your OA much worse.

(Weight loss options are discussed in a different booklet).

How to live well even with OA?

Your health is really your own responsibility.

Along with the appropriate assistance, you should be able to lead a balanced, productive lifestyle even with OA.

OA does not need to become worse in every patient, and also it doesn't necessarily always produce disability.

Self–care

Self-care is an essential part of day-today lifestyle.

This implies you adopt responsibility for your own health and well-being using the assistance from those people associated with your care.

Self-care consists of things that you undertake daily to remain fit and healthy, preserve effective mental and physical wellness, reduce the risk of disease or even injuries, and efficiently manage mild problems as well as long-lasting ailments.

Individuals managing long-lasting

ailments will benefit significantly when they receive assistance with regard to self-care from supportive professionals and carers.

These people can easily live much longer, have less discomfort, uneasiness, misery and exhaustion, enjoy a higher quality of lifestyle and are also much more productive and independent.

Live healthily

A reasonably healthy diet and routine exercising can help maintain muscular tissues and limit your weight, which in turn is useful for OA management and additionally offers various other health advantages.

Be sure to take your prescribed medication

It is crucial to take your medication as recommended, even if you begin feeling much better.

Regular medication can easily assist in preventing discomfort often.

Although if your medications have

been prescribed by a doctor "as needed" (aka PRN) , you possibly will not have to take them in between painful episodes.

If you have any queries or concerns about the treatments you are taking or even undesirable side effects, speak with your professional medical team.

Additionally, it can be of help to read through the information leaflet that is available along with the medication, that will explain all about potential interactions with other medications or supplements.

Consult with your professional medical team if you want to take any "over the counter" alternatives, for example, pain relievers, or perhaps any other natural supplements since these can often interfere with your medication.

Routine Check-ups

Considering that OA is a long-lasting problem, you'll certainly be in frequent contact with your treatment team.

A close alliance with the professionals

should mean that you are able to talk about your disorders or difficulties with them.

The better the team understands your problems, the more they can assist you.

Keeping well

Individuals having a long-lasting disease like OA, is recommended to have an annual flu virus vaccine every autumn in order to protect against flu (influenza).

It's usually suggested they get a pneumococcal vaccination as well.

This is an one-off injection which guards against a severe chest disease called pneumococcal pneumonia.

References

Osteoarthritis: the care and management of osteoarthritis in adults (NICE Guidelines, UK)
http://www.nice.org.uk/guidance/CG59

Osteoarthritis: Diagnosis and Treatment Guidelines (American Family Physicians)
http://www.aafp.org/afp/2012/0101/p49.html

Osteoarthritis Management options in general practice (Australian Family

Physician)
http://www.racgp.org.au/afp/2010/sep
tember/osteoarthritis-%E2%80%93-
management-options-in-general-
practice/

Osteoarthritis in Peripheral Joints -
Diagnosis and Treatment (BC,
Ministry of Health, Canada)
http://www.bcguidelines.ca/guideline
_osteoarthritis.html

Dear Reader,

If you have found the information beneficial, kindly leave behind an honest review of this book on Amazon.

Your thoughts and opinions are highly valued.

Wishing you the very best,

Dr A Mitra